AFIB DIET COOKBOOK FOR SENIORS

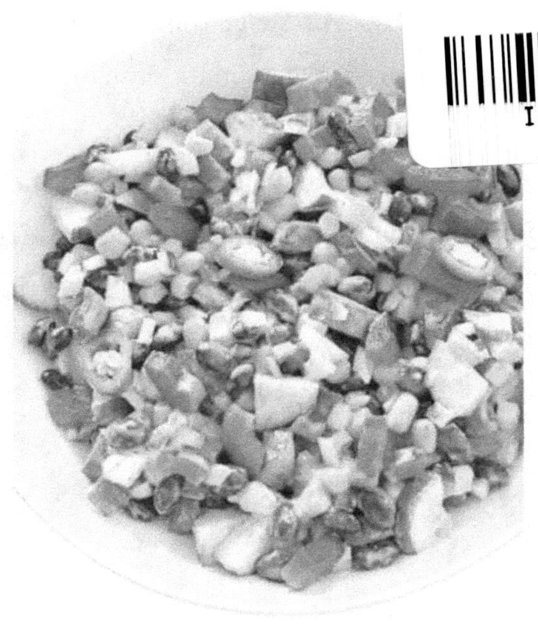

Delicious Recipes for Seniors with AFib

Linda Carlucci

Copyright © 2024 by Linda Carlucci

DISCLAIMER

This cookbook is intended to provide general information and recipes.

The recipes provided in this cookbook are not intended to replace or be a substitute for medical advice from a physician.

The reader should consult a healthcare professional for any specific medical advice, diagnosis or treatment.

Any specific dietary advice provided in this cookbook is not intended to replace or be a substitute for medical advice from a physician.

The author is not responsible or liable for any adverse effects experienced by readers of this cookbook as a result of following the recipes or dietary advice provided.

The author makes no representations or warranties of any kind (express or implied) as to the accuracy, completeness, reliability or suitability of the recipes provided in this cookbook.

The author disclaims any and all liability for any damages arising out of the use or misuse of the recipes provided in this cookbook. The reader must also take care to ensure that the recipes provided in this cookbook are prepared and cooked safely.

The recipes provided in this cookbook are for informational purposes only and should not be used as a substitute for professional medical advice, diagnosis or treatment.

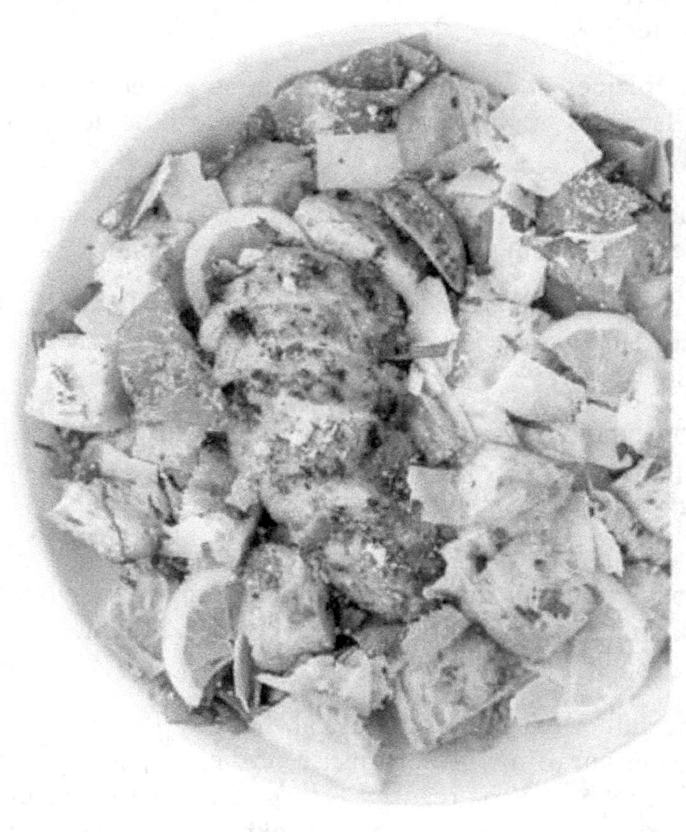

TABLE OF CONTENTS

INTRODUCTION

This cookbook is crafted with care and expertise to provide seniors like you with delicious and nutritious recipes tailored specifically to support their journey in managing atrial fibrillation, a common heart rhythm disorder affecting millions of seniors worldwide.

With a focus on wholesome ingredients, balanced nutrition, and culinary delight, this cookbook aims to help you with AFib to make positive dietary choices that contribute to your overall well-being and heart health.

Atrial fibrillation, often referred to as AFib, is a condition characterized by irregular heartbeats, which can lead to various complications, including stroke and heart failure.

While medication and medical interventions play a vital role in managing AFib, the importance of diet should not be underestimated.

A heart-healthy diet can help you better control your symptoms, reduce the risk of complications, and improve your quality of life.

Recognizing the unique dietary needs and considerations of seniors, this cookbook presents a diverse array of recipes designed to appeal to different tastes and preferences while adhering to the principles of a heart-healthy diet.

Whether you're a seasoned cook or new to the kitchen, each recipe is thoughtfully crafted to be accessible, flavorful, and nourishing, making it easy for you to embrace healthier eating habits without sacrificing taste or enjoyment.

In this book, you'll find a treasure trove of recipes featuring nutrient-rich ingredients, vibrant flavors, and simple cooking techniques.

From comforting soups and stews to satisfying breakfast, hearty mains, and delectable desserts, each dish is carefully curated to support heart health and overall wellness.

As you embark on this culinary journey, I invite you to savor the joy of cooking, nourishing your body, and caring for your heart with each delicious bite. Together, let's embrace the power of food as medicine and embark on a path towards better health and vitality, one wholesome meal at a time.

CHAPTER 1

WHAT IS AFIB?

Atrial fibrillation (AFib) is a common heart rhythm disorder characterized by irregular and often rapid heartbeats.

Normally, the heart's electrical system sends out signals that coordinate the contraction of the upper chambers (atria) and lower chambers (ventricles), allowing blood to flow effectively through the heart and the rest of the body.

However, in AFib, the electrical signals become chaotic, causing the atria to quiver instead of contracting effectively.

This irregular heartbeat can lead to various symptoms, including palpitations, shortness of breath, fatigue, dizziness, and chest discomfort.

Some individuals may not experience any symptoms, making AFib challenging to detect without medical evaluation.

AFib is categorized into several types, including paroxysmal AFib (episodes come and go), persistent AFib (sustained longer episodes), long-standing persistent AFib (continuous

AFib lasting more than a year), and permanent AFib (ongoing, unable to be corrected with treatment).

The condition can occur due to various factors, including age, high blood pressure, heart disease, heart valve disorders, obesity, sleep apnea, thyroid disorders, excessive alcohol consumption, and stimulant use.

Additionally, certain medical conditions such as diabetes and chronic kidney disease can increase the risk of developing AFib.

Complications associated with AFib include an increased risk of stroke due to blood pooling in the atria, which can form clots that travel to the brain.

Other complications include heart failure, which can result from the heart's inability to pump blood effectively over time, and an increased risk of dementia.

Diagnosis typically involves a physical examination, electrocardiogram (ECG or EKG), and possibly other tests such as a Holter monitor, event monitor, echocardiogram, or blood tests.

Treatment aims to control heart rate and rhythm, prevent blood clots, and manage underlying conditions contributing to AFib.

Options may include medications, cardioversion (restoring normal rhythm), catheter ablation, or surgery in certain cases.

Lifestyle modifications such as maintaining a healthy weight, exercising regularly, managing stress, avoiding excessive alcohol and caffeine, and quitting smoking can also help manage AFib and reduce the risk of complications.

Regular monitoring and follow-up with healthcare providers are crucial for managing AFib effectively and minimizing its impact on overall health and quality of life.

THE IMPORTANCE OF A LOW CHOLESTEROL DIET FOR A AFIB CONTROL IN SENIORS

1. **Heart Health:** A low cholesterol diet is essential for seniors with AFib as it supports overall heart health. High cholesterol levels can contribute to plaque

buildup in the arteries, increasing the risk of heart disease and worsening AFib symptoms.

2. **Reduced Risk of Stroke:** By maintaining low cholesterol levels, seniors can lower their risk of stroke, a common complication of AFib. Elevated cholesterol levels can lead to the formation of blood clots, which may travel to the brain and cause a stroke.

3. **Prevention of Atherosclerosis:** Atherosclerosis, the hardening and narrowing of the arteries due to plaque buildup, is a risk factor for AFib. A low cholesterol diet helps prevent the development and progression of atherosclerosis, reducing the strain on the heart.

4. **Improved Blood Flow:** Lowering cholesterol levels promotes better blood flow throughout the body, including the heart. Improved circulation can help reduce the workload on the heart and alleviate symptoms of AFib.

5. **Enhanced Cardiovascular Function:** Seniors with AFib benefit from a low cholesterol diet as it supports optimal cardiovascular function. By reducing cholesterol intake, they can maintain

healthier blood vessels and improve heart function, which is crucial for managing AFib.

6. **Better Response to Medications:** Some medications used to treat AFib, such as statins, work more effectively in individuals with controlled cholesterol levels. Following a low cholesterol diet can enhance the efficacy of these medications and improve AFib control.

7. **Lower Inflammation Levels:** High cholesterol levels are associated with increased inflammation in the body, which can exacerbate AFib symptoms. A low cholesterol diet helps reduce inflammation, leading to better management of AFib and its associated complications.

8. **Stabilized Blood Pressure:** High cholesterol levels can contribute to hypertension, a common risk factor for AFib. By adopting a low cholesterol diet, seniors can help stabilize their blood pressure, reducing the risk of AFib episodes.

9. **Decreased Risk of Arrhythmias:** Elevated cholesterol levels may trigger abnormal heart rhythms, including AFib. By lowering cholesterol

intake, seniors can reduce the likelihood of arrhythmias and improve AFib control.

10. **Support for Weight Management:** Following a low cholesterol diet often involves consuming more fruits, vegetables, and whole grains while limiting saturated and trans fats. This dietary approach supports weight management, which is important for seniors with AFib as obesity can exacerbate symptoms and increase the risk of complications.

11. **Improved Energy Levels:** A low cholesterol diet rich in nutrient-dense foods provides the body with essential vitamins and minerals necessary for energy production. Seniors with AFib may experience improved energy levels and reduced fatigue by adhering to a balanced diet.

12. **Better Overall Health:** Adopting a low cholesterol diet contributes to better overall health and well-being in seniors with AFib. By prioritizing heart-healthy foods, they can reduce their risk of cardiovascular events and improve their quality of life.

13. **Reduced Risk of Diabetes**: High cholesterol levels are associated with insulin resistance and an increased risk of type 2 diabetes, which can worsen AFib symptoms. By controlling cholesterol intake, seniors can lower their risk of developing diabetes and its complications.

14. **Enhanced Nutrient Absorption:** A low cholesterol diet promotes better absorption of essential nutrients, which is particularly important for seniors who may have compromised digestive function. Adequate nutrient intake supports overall health and may help manage AFib more effectively.

15. **Long-Term AFib Management:** Following a low cholesterol diet is essential for long-term management of AFib in seniors. By making dietary changes to control cholesterol levels, they can reduce the frequency and severity of AFib episodes, leading to better outcomes and improved quality of life.

FOODS TO AVOID FOR SENIORS WITH ATRIAL FIBRILLATION

1. **High-Sodium Foods:** Seniors with AFib should avoid high-sodium foods such as processed meats, canned soups, and salty snacks. Excessive sodium intake can contribute to fluid retention and high blood pressure, worsening AFib symptoms.

2. **Fried Foods:** Fried foods, including French fries, fried chicken, and deep-fried snacks, are high in unhealthy fats and calories. These foods can contribute to obesity and heart disease, exacerbating AFib symptoms.

3. **Processed Meats:** Processed meats like bacon, sausage, and deli meats are high in sodium and unhealthy fats. They can increase the risk of heart disease and raise cholesterol levels, making them unsuitable for seniors with AFib.

4. **Sugar-Sweetened Beverages:** Sugary drinks such as soda, sweetened tea, and fruit juices contain high amounts of added sugars. Consuming these beverages can lead to weight gain, insulin resistance,

and inflammation, all of which can worsen AFib symptoms.

5. **Excessive Caffeine:** Seniors with AFib should limit their intake of caffeinated beverages like coffee, tea, and energy drinks. Caffeine can trigger arrhythmias and increase heart rate, potentially exacerbating AFib symptoms.

6. **Alcohol:** Excessive alcohol consumption can trigger AFib episodes and increase the risk of complications such as stroke. Seniors with AFib should limit their alcohol intake or avoid it altogether to better manage their condition.

7. **High-Fat Dairy Products:** High-fat dairy products like whole milk, high-fat cheese, and ice cream, which can raise cholesterol levels and contribute to heart disease. Seniors with AFib should opt for low-fat or non-fat dairy alternatives.

8. **Processed Foods:** Processed foods such as packaged snacks, frozen meals, and instant noodles often contain high amounts of sodium, unhealthy fats, and additives. These ingredients can negatively impact

heart health and should be avoided by seniors with AFib.

9. **Excessively Spicy Foods:** Spicy foods can stimulate the heart and increase heart rate, potentially triggering AFib episodes. Seniors with AFib should moderate their intake of spicy foods to avoid exacerbating their symptoms.

10. **Excessive Red Meat:** While lean cuts of red meat can be part of a healthy diet, excessive consumption may increase the risk of heart disease and worsen AFib symptoms. Seniors with AFib should limit their intake of red meat and opt for leaner protein sources like poultry, fish, and plant-based proteins.

11. **High-Cholesterol Foods:** Foods high in cholesterol, such as egg yolks, organ meats, and full-fat dairy products, can raise cholesterol levels and increase the risk of heart disease. Seniors with AFib should avoid or limit their intake of these foods to support heart health.

12. **Trans Fats:** Trans fats are found in fried foods, baked goods, and margarine and can raise LDL (bad) cholesterol levels while lowering HDL (good)

cholesterol levels. Seniors with AFib should avoid foods containing trans fats to reduce their risk of heart disease.

13. **Excessive Salt Substitutes:** Some salt substitutes contain high amounts of potassium, which can be harmful to individuals with certain medical conditions, including kidney disease and heart failure. Seniors with AFib should avoid excessive use of salt substitutes and consult their healthcare provider for guidance.

14. **High-Glycemic Index Foods:** Foods with a high glycemic index, such as white bread, white rice, and sugary cereals, can cause rapid spikes in blood sugar levels. These fluctuations may contribute to inflammation and increase the risk of heart disease in seniors with AFib.

15. **Fast Food:** Fast food items like burgers, fries, and pizza are typically high in unhealthy fats, sodium, and calories. Regular consumption of fast food can contribute to obesity, high blood pressure, and heart disease, all of which can exacerbate AFib symptoms. Seniors with AFib should avoid fast food and

prioritize home-cooked meals made with fresh, whole ingredients.

HEALTHY FLAVOR ALTERNATIVES TO ALTERNATIVES TO REPLACE SODIUM IN YOUR DIET

1. **Herbs:** Fresh or dried herbs such as basil, thyme, rosemary, and oregano can add flavor to dishes without the need for salt. Use them generously in soups, salads, marinades, and sauces to enhance taste.

2. **Citrus:** Citrus fruits like lemon, lime, and orange provide a burst of flavor and acidity that can mimic the taste of salt. Squeeze fresh citrus juice over vegetables, fish, or poultry before cooking or use zest to add depth to dishes.

3. **Vinegar:** Vinegar, whether balsamic, apple cider, or red wine vinegar, adds tanginess and complexity to recipes without the need for salt. Use it in dressings, marinades, and sauces to enhance flavor.

4. **Spices:** A wide variety of spices, such as cumin, paprika, chili powder, and curry powder, can add

depth and heat to dishes without relying on salt. Experiment with different spice blends to create flavorful meals.

5. **Garlic and Onion:** Fresh garlic and onion are aromatic ingredients that can elevate the taste of any dish. Sauté them in olive oil as a base for soups, stews, and stir-fries, or roast them with vegetables for added flavor.

6. **Ginger:** Fresh ginger adds warmth and spice to both savory and sweet dishes. Grate it into marinades, dressings, and sauces, or use it to infuse flavor into soups and stir-fries.

7. **Mustard:** Dijon mustard and whole-grain mustard provide a tangy flavor that can enhance sandwiches, salads, and sauces. Use them as a condiment or incorporate them into marinades and glazes.

8. **Fresh Herbs:** Instead of relying on salt, use fresh herbs like parsley, cilantro, and dill to brighten up dishes. Sprinkle chopped herbs over cooked meals or use them as a garnish for added flavor.

9. **Miso Paste:** Miso paste, made from fermented soybeans, adds depth and umami flavor to dishes.

Use it as a base for soups, dressings, and sauces, or mix it with vinegar and oil for a flavorful marinade.

10. **Nutritional Yeast:** Nutritional yeast has a cheesy, nutty flavor that can enhance the taste of various dishes. Sprinkle it over popcorn, pasta, or roasted vegetables for a savory twist without the need for salt.

11. **Tamari or Soy Sauce:** Tamari or low-sodium soy sauce adds a rich, savory flavor to dishes without the high sodium content of traditional table salt. Use it sparingly in stir-fries, marinades, and dipping sauces.

12. **Homemade Stocks:** Make homemade stocks or broths using vegetables, herbs, and aromatics to infuse dishes with flavor. Use these stocks as a base for soups, stews, and sauces instead of relying on store-bought broths that may be high in sodium.

13. **Coconut Aminos:** Coconut aminos are a salty-sweet alternative to soy sauce that works well in Asian-inspired dishes. Use them in stir-fries, marinades, and dressings for a lower-sodium flavor boost.

14. **Lemon Pepper Seasoning**: Lemon pepper seasoning blends tangy citrus with spicy black

pepper for a versatile flavor enhancer. Use it to season poultry, fish, vegetables, or salads for added zest without the need for salt.

15. **Homemade Spice Blends:** Create your own salt-free spice blends using a combination of herbs, spices, and aromatics. Experiment with different flavor profiles, such as Italian, Cajun, or Mediterranean, to customize dishes to your taste preferences while reducing sodium intake.

EFFECTIVE STRESS REDUCTION STRATEGIES FOR SENIORS WITH AFIB

1. **Deep Breathing Exercises:** Deep breathing techniques can help seniors relax and reduce stress, which in turn can help manage AFib symptoms.

2. **Mindfulness Meditation**: Practicing mindfulness meditation can help seniors focus on the present moment, reducing anxiety and stress associated with AFib.

3. **Yoga:** Gentle yoga poses and stretches can help seniors improve flexibility, reduce muscle tension, and promote relaxation.

4. **Tai Chi:** Tai Chi is a low-impact exercise that combines gentle movements and deep breathing, promoting relaxation and reducing stress levels.

5. **Progressive Muscle Relaxation:** This technique involves tensing and relaxing different muscle groups in the body, helping seniors release tension and stress.

6. **Guided Imagery:** Guided imagery involves visualizing peaceful and calming scenes, helping seniors relax and alleviate stress.

7. **Adequate Sleep:** Ensuring seniors get enough restful sleep is crucial for managing stress and reducing AFib symptoms.

8. **Regular Exercise:** Engaging in regular physical activity can help seniors reduce stress, improve cardiovascular health, and manage AFib symptoms.

9. **Healthy Diet:** Eating a balanced diet rich in fruits, vegetables, whole grains, and lean proteins can help seniors manage stress and maintain overall health.

10. **Social Support:** Connecting with friends, family, or support groups can provide seniors with emotional support and reduce feelings of stress and isolation.

11. **Limiting Caffeine and Alcohol:** Consuming excessive caffeine and alcohol can exacerbate AFib symptoms and increase stress levels, so seniors should limit their intake.

12. **Setting Realistic Goals:** Seniors should set achievable goals and prioritize tasks to avoid feeling overwhelmed, which can contribute to stress.

13. **Prioritizing Relaxation:** Making time for relaxation activities such as reading, listening to music, or enjoying hobbies can help seniors unwind and reduce stress levels.

14. **Breathing Techniques:** Practicing breathing exercises such as diaphragmatic breathing or square breathing can help seniors calm their nervous system and reduce stress.

15. **Seeking Professional Help:** If stress becomes overwhelming, seniors should not hesitate to seek support from healthcare professionals, therapists, or

counselors who can provide coping strategies and support tailored to their needs.

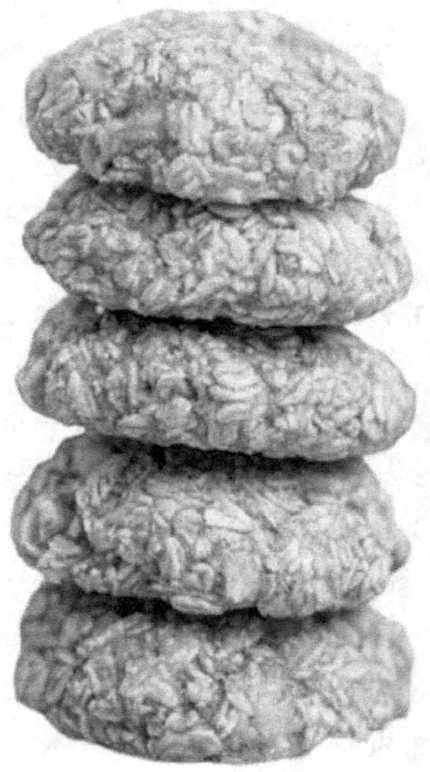

CHAPTER 2

14-DAY MEAL PLAN

DAY 1

BREAKFAST: Spinach and Mushroom Egg White Omelet

LUNCH: Quinoa and Vegetable Stir-Fry

DINNER: Grilled Chicken Breast with Roasted Vegetables

DAY 2

BREAKFAST: Chia Seed Pudding with Mixed Fruit

LUNCH: Turkey and Avocado Wrap with Whole Wheat Tortilla

DINNER: Turkey and Vegetable Chili

DAY 3

BREAKFAST: Quinoa Breakfast Bowl with Spinach and Poached Egg

LUNCH: Lentil Soup with Spinach

DINNER: Lemon Herb Roasted Chicken with Steamed Broccoli

DAY 4

BREAKFAST: Oatmeal with Fresh Berries and Almonds

LUNCH: Mediterranean Chickpea Salad with Feta Cheese

DINNER: Grilled Cod with Mango Salsa

DAY 5

BREAKFAST: Low-fat Greek Yogurt Parfait with Honey and Walnuts

LUNCH: Grilled Chicken Caesar Salad with Light Dressing

DINNER: Spinach and Feta Stuffed Bell Peppers

DAY 6

BREAKFAST: Low-fat Cottage Cheese Pancakes with Blueberry Compote

LUNCH: Veggie and Hummus Sandwich on Whole Grain Bread

DINNER: Shrimp and Vegetable Skewers with Brown Rice

DAY 7

BREAKFAST: Banana Almond Smoothie with Flaxseeds

LUNCH: Spinach and Mushroom Omelet with Whole Wheat Toast

DINNER: Baked Tilapia with Herb Crust

DAY 8

BREAKFAST: Buckwheat Pancakes with Greek Yogurt and Raspberry Sauce

LUNCH: Roasted Vegetable Quinoa Bowl with Balsamic Glaze

DINNER: Eggplant Parmesan with Whole Wheat Pasta

DAY 9

BREAKFAST: Veggie Breakfast Burrito with Black Beans and Salsa

LUNCH: Shrimp and Vegetable Stir-Fry with Brown Rice

DINNER: Turkey Meatballs with Marinara Sauce and Zucchini Noodles

DAY 10

BREAKFAST: Overnight Oats with Apple Cinnamon and Pecans

LUNCH: Black Bean and Corn Salad with Lime Dressing

DINNER: Baked Chicken Thighs with Sweet Potatoes and Brussels Sprouts

DAY 11

BREAKFAST: Spinach and Mushroom Egg White Omelet

LUNCH: Quinoa and Vegetable Stir-Fry

DINNER: Grilled Chicken Breast with Roasted Vegetables

DAY 12

BREAKFAST: Chia Seed Pudding with Mixed Fruit

LUNCH: Turkey and Avocado Wrap with Whole Wheat Tortilla

DINNER: Turkey and Vegetable Chili

DAY 13

BREAKFAST: Quinoa Breakfast Bowl with Spinach and Poached Egg

LUNCH: Lentil Soup with Spinach

DINNER: Lemon Herb Roasted Chicken with Steamed Broccoli

DAY 14

BREAKFAST: Oatmeal with Fresh Berries and Almonds

LUNCH: Mediterranean Chickpea Salad with Feta Cheese

DINNER: Grilled Cod with Mango Salsa

DAY 15

BREAKFAST: Greek Yogurt Parfait with Honey and Walnuts

LUNCH: Grilled Chicken Caesar Salad with Light Dressing

DINNER: Spinach and Feta Stuffed Bell Peppers

CHAPTER 3

NUTRITIOUS RECIP1ES FOR AFIB DIET COOKBOOK

BREAKFAST

Spinach and Mushroom Egg White Omelet

Preparation Time: 15 minutes

Serves: 2

Calories: 90g **Sodium:** 50mg **Fats:** 5g **Carbs:** 4g **Cholesterol:** 0mg **Fiber:** 1g

Ingredients:

4 egg whites

1 cup fresh spinach, chopped

½ cup mushrooms, sliced

1 tablespoon olive oil

2 tablespoons diced onions

1 clove garlic, minced

¼ teaspoon black pepper

¼ teaspoon dried thyme

Cooking spray

Method of Preparation:

1. In a non-stick skillet, heat olive oil over medium heat.
2. Add diced onions and minced garlic to the skillet, sautéing until translucent.
3. Add sliced mushrooms and chopped spinach to the skillet, cooking until the vegetables are tender.
4. In a separate bowl, whisk the egg whites until frothy.
5. Season with black pepper and dried thyme.
6. Coat the skillet with cooking spray and pour in the egg whites, swirling to evenly distribute.
7. Cook the egg whites until set, then add the cooked vegetables on one half of the omelet.
8. Gently fold the other half of the omelet over the vegetables.

Chia Seed Pudding with Mixed Fruit

Preparation Time: 5 minutes

Serves: 2

Calories: 150g **Sodium:** 40mg **Fats:** 7g **Carbs:** 9g
Cholesterol: 0mg **Fiber:** 9g

Ingredients:

¼ cup chia seeds

1 cup unsweetened almond milk

½ teaspoon vanilla extract

1 tablespoon honey (or maple syrup)

½ cup mixed fruits (such as berries, sliced banana, and kiwi)

Method of Preparation:

1. In a mixing bowl, combine chia seeds, almond milk, vanilla extract, and honey.
2. Stir well to combine.
3. Cover the bowl and refrigerate for at least 4 hours or overnight, allowing the chia seeds to absorb the liquid and thicken.

4. Once the chia pudding has set, divide it into serving bowls.

5. Top each bowl with mixed fruits.

Quinoa Breakfast Bowl with Spinach and Poached Egg

Preparation Time: 20 minutes

Serves: 2

Calories: 320g **Sodium:** 40mg **Fats:** 16g **Carbs:** 10g **Cholesterol:** 50mg **Fiber:** 9g

Ingredients:

1 cup cooked quinoa

1 cup fresh spinach

2 large eggs

½ avocado, sliced

1 tablespoon lemon juice

1 teaspoon olive oil

¼ teaspoon black pepper

Method of Preparation:

1. In a small saucepan, bring water to a simmer.
2. Crack each egg into a separate small bowl.
3. Gently slide the eggs, one at a time, into the simmering water.
4. Poach for 3-4 minutes until the whites are set but the yolks are still runny.
5. While the eggs are poaching, heat olive oil in a skillet over medium heat.
6. Add fresh spinach and sauté until wilted.
7. In a mixing bowl, toss cooked quinoa with lemon juice and black pepper.
8. Divide the seasoned quinoa into serving bowls.
9. Top each bowl with sautéed spinach, sliced avocado, and a poached egg.

Oatmeal with Fresh Berries and Almonds

Preparation Time: 10 minutes

Serves: 2

Calories: 250g **Sodium:** 5mg **Fats:** 8g **Carbs:** 38g **Cholesterol:** 0mg **Fiber:** 7g

Ingredients:

1 cup old-fashioned oats

2 cups water

½ cup fresh mixed berries (such as strawberries, blueberries, and raspberries)

2 tablespoons sliced almonds

1 tablespoon honey (optional)

Method of Preparation:

1. In a saucepan, bring water to a boil.
2. Stir in the oats and reduce the heat to low.
3. Cook for 5-7 minutes, stirring occasionally, until the oats are tender and creamy.
4. Divide the cooked oatmeal into serving bowls.
5. Top each bowl with fresh mixed berries and sliced almonds.
6. Drizzle honey over the oatmeal, if desired.

Low-Fat Greek Yogurt Parfait with Honey and Walnuts

Preparation Time: 5 minutes

Serves: 2

Calories: 130g **Sodium:** 40mg **Fats:** 10g **Carbs:** 4g **Cholesterol:** 5mg **Fiber:** 3g

Ingredients:

1 cup low-fat Greek yogurt (unsweetened)

½ cup mixed fresh berries (such as strawberries, blueberries, and raspberries)

2 tablespoons chopped walnuts

1 tablespoon honey

Method of Preparation:

1. In serving glasses or bowls, layer Greek yogurt, mixed fresh berries, and chopped walnuts.
2. Drizzle honey over the top of each parfait.
3. Repeat the layers until all ingredients are used.

Low-Fat Cottage Cheese Pancakes with Blueberry Compote

Preparation Time: 20 minutes

Serves: 2

Calories: 120g **Sodium:** 40mg **Fats:** 6g **Carbs:** 8g **Cholesterol:** 50mg **Fiber:** 6g

Ingredients for Pancakes:

1 cup cottage cheese (low-fat)

2 large eggs

½ cup whole wheat flour

1 teaspoon baking powder

1 tablespoon honey

½ teaspoon vanilla extract

Cooking spray or olive oil for cooking

Ingredients for Blueberry Compote:

1 cup fresh or frozen blueberries

2 tablespoons water

1 tablespoon honey

½ teaspoon lemon juice

Method of Preparation:

1. In a blender or food processor, combine cottage cheese, eggs, whole wheat flour, baking powder, honey, and vanilla extract.
2. Blend until smooth.
3. Heat a non-stick skillet or griddle over medium heat and lightly coat with cooking spray or olive oil.
4. Pour about ¼ cup of batter onto the skillet for each pancake.
5. Cook until bubbles form on the surface, then flip and cook until golden brown on both sides.
6. Meanwhile, in a small saucepan, combine blueberries, water, honey, and lemon juice.
7. Cook over medium heat until the blueberries burst and the mixture thickens, stirring occasionally.
8. Serve the pancakes with the blueberry compote on top.

Banana Almond Smoothie with Flaxseeds

Preparation Time: 5 minutes

Serves: 2

Calories: 150g **Sodium:** 150mg **Fats:** 5g **Carbs:** 7g **Cholesterol:** 0mg **Fiber:** 6g

Ingredients:

1 ripe banana

1 cup unsweetened almond milk

2 tablespoons almond butter

1 tablespoon flaxseeds

½ teaspoon cinnamon

Ice cubes (optional)

Method of Preparation:

1. In a blender, combine banana, almond milk, almond butter, flaxseeds, and cinnamon.
2. Add ice cubes if desired for a colder smoothie.

3. Blend until smooth and creamy.

4. Pour into glasses and serve immediately.

Buckwheat Pancakes with Greek Yogurt and Raspberry Sauce

Preparation Time: 20 minutes

Serves: 2

Calories: 100g **Sodium:** 30mg **Fats:** 5g **Carbs:** 20g **Cholesterol:** 55mg **Fiber:** 9g

Ingredients for Pancakes:

1 cup buckwheat flour

1 teaspoon baking powder

½ teaspoon baking soda

1 tablespoon honey

1 large egg

1 cup unsweetened almond milk (or any milk of choice)

Cooking spray or olive oil for cooking

Ingredients for Raspberry Sauce:

1 cup fresh or frozen raspberries

2 tablespoons water

1 tablespoon honey

Method of Preparation:

1. In a mixing bowl, combine buckwheat flour, baking powder, baking soda, honey, egg, and almond milk.
2. Mix until smooth.
3. Heat a non-stick skillet or griddle over medium heat and lightly coat with cooking spray or olive oil.
4. Pour about ¼ cup of batter onto the skillet for each pancake.
5. Cook until bubbles form on the surface, then flip and cook until golden brown on both sides.
6. Meanwhile, in a small saucepan, combine raspberries, water, and honey.
7. Cook over medium heat until the raspberries break down and the mixture thickens, stirring occasionally.
8. Serve the pancakes with a dollop of Greek yogurt and raspberry sauce on top.

Veggie Breakfast Burrito with Black Beans and Salsa

Preparation Time: 15 minutes

Serves: 2

Calories: 150g **Sodium:** 40mg **Fats:** 5g **Carbs:** 6g **Cholesterol:** 0mg **Fiber:** 15g

Ingredients:

2 large whole wheat tortillas

1 cup black beans, cooked

1 cup bell peppers, diced

1 cup tomatoes, diced

1 cup spinach leaves

½ cup red onion, diced

½ cup salsa (low-sodium)

½ teaspoon cumin

¼ teaspoon paprika

Cooking spray or olive oil for cooking

Method of Preparation:

1. In a skillet, heat cooking spray or olive oil over medium heat.
2. Add diced bell peppers and red onion, sautéing until softened.
3. Add black beans, diced tomatoes, spinach leaves, cumin, and paprika to the skillet.
4. Cook until the spinach wilts and the mixture are heated through.
5. Warm the whole wheat tortillas in the microwave or on a skillet for a few seconds to make them pliable.
6. Divide the vegetable and black bean mixture evenly between the tortillas.
7. Top each burrito with salsa.
8. Roll up the tortillas tightly to form burritos, tucking in the sides as you roll.
9. Serve immediately or wrap in foil for a portable breakfast option.

Overnight Oats with Apple Cinnamon and Pecans

Preparation Time: 5 minutes

Serves: 2

Calories: 180g **Sodium:** 70mg **Fats:** 10g **Carbs:** 45g
Cholesterol: 0mg **Fiber:** 7g

Ingredients:

1 cup old-fashioned oats

1 cup unsweetened almond milk

1 apple, diced

1 tablespoon honey or maple syrup

½ teaspoon cinnamon

2 tablespoons chopped pecans

Method of Preparation:

1. In a jar or container with a lid, combine old-fashioned oats, almond milk, diced apple, honey or maple syrup, and cinnamon.
2. Stir well to combine.
3. Cover the jar or container and refrigerate overnight, allowing the oats to soften and absorb the liquid.
4. In the morning, give the oats a stir and top with chopped pecans before serving.

5. Enjoy cold or warm by heating in the microwave for a few seconds.

LUNCH

Quinoa and Vegetable Stir-Fry

Preparation Time: 30 minutes

Serves: 2

Calories: 180g **Sodium:** 40mg **Fats:** 8g **Carbs:** 5g **Cholesterol:** 0mg **Fiber:** 11g

Ingredients:

1 cup quinoa, rinsed

2 cups water or vegetable broth

1 tablespoon olive oil

2 cloves garlic, minced

1 cup bell peppers, sliced

1/2 cup broccoli florets

1 cup carrots, julienned

1 cup snap peas

½ cup low-sodium soy sauce

1 tablespoon rice vinegar

1 tablespoon honey or maple syrup

1 teaspoon ginger, grated

¼ teaspoon red pepper flakes (optional)

Sesame seeds for garnish (optional)

Chopped green onions for garnish (optional)

Method of Preparation:

1. In a saucepan, combine quinoa and water or vegetable broth.
2. Bring to a boil, then reduce heat to low, cover, and simmer for 15-20 minutes, or until the quinoa is cooked and the liquid is absorbed.
3. Fluff with a fork and set aside.
4. In a large skillet or wok, heat olive oil over medium-high heat.
5. Add minced garlic and cook for 1 minute, or until fragrant.

6. Add sliced bell peppers, broccoli florets, julienned carrots, and snap peas to the skillet.

7. Stir-fry for 5-7 minutes, or until the vegetables are tender-crisp.

8. In a small bowl, whisk together low-sodium soy sauce, rice vinegar, honey or maple syrup, grated ginger, and red pepper flakes, if using.

9. Pour the sauce over the vegetables in the skillet.

10. Add cooked quinoa and toss to coat everything evenly with the sauce.

11. Cook for an additional 2-3 minutes, or until heated through.

12. Garnish with sesame seeds and chopped green onions, if desired.

Turkey and Avocado Wrap with Whole Wheat Tortilla

Preparation Time: 10 minutes

Serves: 2

Calories: 150g **Sodium:** 50mg **Fats:** 14g **Carbs:** 4g **Cholesterol:** 30mg **Fiber:** 10g

Ingredients:

2 large whole wheat tortillas

4 slices turkey breast (low-sodium)

1 ripe avocado, sliced

1 cup mixed greens

½ cup cherry tomatoes, halved

¼ cup cucumber, sliced

2 tablespoons hummus

Method of Preparation:

1. Lay each whole wheat tortilla flat on a clean surface.
2. Spread 1 tablespoon of hummus onto each tortilla.
3. Layer 2 slices of turkey breast, sliced avocado, mixed greens, cherry tomatoes, and sliced cucumber onto each tortilla.
4. Roll up the tortillas tightly to form wraps, tucking in the sides as you roll.
5. Slice each wrap in half diagonally.
6. Serve immediately or wrap in foil for a portable lunch option.

Lentil Soup with Spinach

Preparation Time: 45 minutes

Serves: 2

Calories: 120g **Sodium:** 40mg **Fats:** 5g **Carbs:** 5g
Cholesterol: 0mg **Fiber:** 20g

Ingredients:

1 cup dried green lentils, rinsed

4 cups vegetable broth

1 tablespoon olive oil

1 onion, diced

2 cloves garlic, minced

1 carrot, diced

1 celery stalk, diced

1 teaspoon dried thyme

1 teaspoon dried oregano

1 bay leaf

2 cups fresh spinach leaves

Chopped fresh parsley for garnish (optional)

Method of Preparation:

1. In a large pot, heat olive oil over medium heat.
2. Add diced onion, minced garlic, diced carrot, and diced celery.
3. Sauté for 5-7 minutes, or until the vegetables are softened.
4. Add rinsed green lentils, vegetable broth, dried thyme, dried oregano, and bay leaf to the pot.
5. Bring to a boil, then reduce heat to low, cover, and simmer for 25-30 minutes, or until the lentils are tender.
6. Stir in fresh spinach leaves.
7. Cook for an additional 5 minutes, or until the spinach wilts.
8. Remove the bay leaf before serving.
9. Ladle the soup into bowls and garnish with chopped fresh parsley, if desired.

Mediterranean Chickpea Salad with Feta Cheese

Preparation Time: 15 minutes

Serves: 2

Calories: 120g **Sodium:** 50mg **Fats:** 18g **Carbs:** 30g **Cholesterol:** 15mg **Fiber:** 9g

Ingredients:

1 can (15 oz) chickpeas, drained and rinsed

1 bell pepper, diced

1 cucumber, diced

1/4 cup red onion, finely chopped

1/4 cup Kalamata olives, pitted and halved

2 tablespoons fresh parsley, chopped

2 tablespoons extra virgin olive oil

1 tablespoon lemon juice

1 teaspoon dried oregano

1/4 cup crumbled feta cheese

Method of Preparation:

1. In a large mixing bowl, combine the chickpeas, bell pepper, cucumber, red onion, Kalamata olives, and parsley.
2. In a small bowl, whisk together the extra virgin olive oil, lemon juice, dried oregano, salt, and black pepper to make the dressing.
3. Pour the dressing over the salad ingredients and toss until evenly coated.
4. Sprinkle the crumbled feta cheese over the top of the salad.
5. Serve chilled or at room temperature.

Grilled Chicken Caesar Salad with Light Dressing

Preparation Time: 20 minutes

Serves: 2

Calories: 180g **Sodium:** 50mg **Fats:** 10g **Carbs:** 15g
Cholesterol: 40mg **Fiber:** 5g

Ingredients:

2 boneless, skinless chicken breasts

4 cups romaine lettuce, chopped

1/4 cup grated Swiss cheese

1/4 cup whole wheat croutons

Light Caesar dressing (homemade or store-bought, low-sodium)

Method of Preparation:

1. Preheat the grill to medium-high heat.
2. Season the chicken breasts with desired spice
3. Grill the chicken breasts for 6-8 minutes per side, or until cooked through and no longer pink in the center.
4. Remove from the grill and let rest for a few minutes before slicing.
5. In a large salad bowl, combine the chopped romaine lettuce, grated Swiss cheese, and whole wheat croutons.
6. Add the sliced grilled chicken to the salad bowl.
7. Drizzle with light Caesar dressing and toss until evenly coated.

Veggie and Hummus Sandwich on Whole Grain Bread

Preparation Time: 10 minutes

Serves: 2

Calories: 120g **Sodium:** 40mg **Fats:** 15g **Carbs:** 40g

Cholesterol: 0mg **Fiber:** 12g

Ingredients:

4 slices whole grain bread

1/2 cup hummus (homemade or store-bought, low-sodium)

1/2 cucumber, thinly sliced

1/2 red bell pepper, thinly sliced

1/2 avocado, thinly sliced

1/4 cup alfalfa sprouts

Method of Preparation:

1. Spread hummus evenly onto each slice of whole grain bread.

2. Layer cucumber slices, red bell pepper slices, avocado slices, and alfalfa sprouts onto two slices of bread.

3. Season with desired spice.

4. Top with the remaining slices of bread to form sandwiches.

5. Slice in half diagonally.

6. Serve immediately or wrap in foil for a portable lunch option.

Spinach and Mushroom Omelet with Whole Wheat Toast

Preparation Time: 15 minutes

Serves: 2

Calories: 120g **Sodium:** 40mg **Fats:** 17g **Carbs:** 22g **Cholesterol:** 40mg **Fiber:** 5g

Ingredients:

4 large eggs

1 cup fresh spinach leaves

1/2 cup sliced mushrooms

2 tablespoons diced onion

1 tablespoon olive oil

2 slices whole wheat bread, toasted

Method of Preparation:

1. In a mixing bowl, beat the eggs until well combined. Add up some seasoning.
2. Heat olive oil in a non-stick skillet over medium heat.
3. Add diced onion and sliced mushrooms, and cook until softened.
4. Add fresh spinach leaves to the skillet and cook until wilted.
5. Pour the beaten eggs over the vegetables in the skillet.
6. Cook until the omelet is set, then fold it in half.
7. Transfer the omelet to a plate and serve with whole wheat toast.

Roasted Vegetable Quinoa Bowl with Balsamic Glaze

Preparation Time: 30 minutes

Serves: 2

Calories: 180g **Sodium:** 50mg **Fats:** 8g **Carbs:** 45g **Cholesterol:** 0mg **Fiber:** 7g

Ingredients:

1 cup cooked quinoa

1 cup mixed vegetables (such as bell peppers, zucchini, and cherry tomatoes)

1 tablespoon olive oil

2 tablespoons balsamic glaze

Fresh basil leaves for garnish (optional)

A pinch of salt and pepper

Method of Preparation:

1. Preheat the oven to 400°F (200°C).
2. Toss mixed vegetables with olive oil, a pinch of salt and pepper on a baking sheet.
3. Roast the vegetables in the preheated oven for 20-25 minutes, or until tender and slightly caramelized.
4. Divide cooked quinoa among serving bowls.
5. Top with roasted vegetables.

6. Drizzle balsamic glaze over the quinoa and vegetables.

7. Garnish with fresh basil leaves, if desired.

Shrimp and Vegetable Stir-Fry with Brown Rice

Preparation Time: 20 minutes

Serves: 2

Calories: 180g **Sodium:** 50mg **Fats:** 10g **Carbs:** 45g **Cholesterol:** 20mg **Fiber:** 6g

Ingredients:

1 lb. shrimp, peeled and deveined

2 cups mixed vegetables (such as bell peppers, broccoli, and snap peas), sliced

2 cloves garlic, minced

1 tablespoon ginger, grated

2 tablespoons low-sodium soy sauce

1 tablespoon hoisin sauce

1 tablespoon sesame oil

2 cups cooked brown rice

1 tablespoon olive oil

Sesame seeds for garnish (optional)

Chopped green onions for garnish (optional)

Method of Preparation:

1. Heat olive oil in a large skillet or wok over medium-high heat.
2. Add minced garlic and grated ginger to the skillet, and cook until fragrant.
3. Add shrimp to the skillet and cook until pink and cooked through.
4. Remove shrimp from the skillet and set aside.
5. In the same skillet, add sliced mixed vegetables and stir-fry until tender-crisp.
6. Return the cooked shrimp to the skillet.
7. In a small bowl, whisk together low-sodium soy sauce, hoisin sauce, and sesame oil.
8. Pour the sauce over the shrimp and vegetables in the skillet.

9. Cook for an additional 1-2 minutes, stirring to coat everything evenly with the sauce.

10. Serve the shrimp and vegetable stir-fry over cooked brown rice.

11. Garnish with sesame seeds and chopped green onions, if desired.

Black Bean and Corn Salad with Lime Dressing

Preparation Time: 10 minutes

Serves: 2

Calories: 180g **Sodium:** 50mg **Fats:** 7g **Carbs:** 45g **Cholesterol:** 0mg **Fiber:** 10g

Ingredients:

1 can (15 oz) black beans, drained and rinsed

1 cup corn kernels (fresh, canned, or frozen)

1/4 cup red bell pepper, diced

1/4 cup red onion, finely chopped

1/4 cup cilantro, chopped

1 tablespoon olive oil

2 tablespoons lime juice

1 teaspoon honey

1/2 teaspoon cumin

Avocado slices for serving (optional)

Method of Preparation:

1. In a large mixing bowl, combine black beans, corn kernels, diced red bell pepper, chopped red onion, and chopped cilantro.

2. In a small bowl, whisk together olive oil, lime juice, honey, and desired spice to make the dressing.

3. Pour the dressing over the black bean and corn mixture, and toss until evenly coated.

4. Serve the salad chilled or at room temperature.

5. Garnish with avocado slices, if desired.

DINNER

Grilled Chicken Breast with Roasted Vegetables

Preparation Time: 25 minutes

Serves: 2

Calories: 200g **Sodium:** 40mg **Fats:** 12g **Carbs:** 15g
Cholesterol: 80mg **Fiber:** 5g

Ingredients:

2 boneless, skinless chicken breasts

2 cups mixed vegetables (such as bell peppers, zucchini, and carrots), sliced

2 tablespoons olive oil

2 cloves garlic, minced

1 teaspoon Italian seasoning

Method of Preparation:

1. Preheat the grill to medium-high heat.

2. Season the chicken breasts with minced garlic, Italian seasoning and black pepper if desired.

3. Brush the chicken breasts and mixed vegetables with olive oil.

4. Place the chicken breasts and mixed vegetables on the grill.

5. Grill the chicken breasts for 6-8 minutes per side, or until cooked through and no longer pink in the center.

6. Grill the mixed vegetables until tender and slightly charred, flipping occasionally.

7. Remove the chicken breasts and mixed vegetables from the grill.

8. Serve the grilled chicken breasts with roasted vegetables on the side.

Turkey and Vegetable Chili

Preparation Time: 35 minutes

Serves: 2

Calories: 120g **Sodium:** 40mg **Fats:** 10g **Carbs:** 30g **Cholesterol:** 60mg **Fiber:** 8g

Ingredients:

1 lb. ground turkey

1 onion, diced

2 cloves garlic, minced

1 bell pepper, diced

1 zucchini, diced

1 can (15 oz) diced tomatoes

1 can (15 oz) black beans, drained and rinsed

1 cup corn kernels (fresh, canned, or frozen)

2 cups low-sodium chicken broth

2 tablespoons chili powder

1 teaspoon cumin

Chopped fresh cilantro for garnish (optional)

Greek yogurt for serving (optional)

Method of Preparation:

1. In a large pot, cook ground turkey over medium heat until browned and cooked through.

2. Add diced onion and minced garlic to the pot, and cook until softened.

3. Add diced bell pepper and diced zucchini to the pot, and cook until tender.

4. Stir in diced tomatoes, black beans, corn kernels, low-sodium chicken broth, chili powder, and cumin.

5. Bring the chili to a boil, then reduce heat to low and simmer for 20-25 minutes, stirring occasionally.

6. Season with desired low sodium spice.

7. Serve the turkey and vegetable chili hot, garnished with chopped fresh cilantro and a dollop of Greek yogurt, if desired.

Lemon Herb Roasted Chicken with Steamed Broccoli

Preparation Time: 30 minutes

Serves: 2

Calories: 120g **Sodium:** 20mg **Fats:** 15g **Carbs:** 10g **Cholesterol:** 40mg **Fiber:** 4g

Ingredients:

2 boneless, skinless chicken breasts

2 tablespoons olive oil

1 lemon, juiced and zested

2 cloves garlic, minced

1 teaspoon dried thyme

1 teaspoon dried rosemary

2 cups broccoli florets

Method of Preparation:

1. Preheat the oven to 400°F (200°C).
2. In a small bowl, whisk together olive oil, lemon juice, lemon zest, minced garlic, dried thyme, dried rosemary and desired spices.
3. Place chicken breasts in a baking dish and pour the lemon herb mixture over them, ensuring they are evenly coated.
4. Bake in the preheated oven for 20-25 minutes, or until the chicken is cooked through and juices run clear.
5. While the chicken is baking, steam broccoli florets until tender.

6. Serve the lemon herb roasted chicken with steamed broccoli on the side.

Grilled Cod with Mango Salsa

Preparation Time: 20 minutes

Serves: 2

Calories: 180g **Sodium:** 20mg **Fats:** 10g **Carbs:** 25g **Cholesterol:** 50mg **Fiber:** 5g

Ingredients:

2 cod fillets

1 tablespoon olive oil

1 tablespoon Italian spice

1 mango, diced

1/4 red onion, finely chopped

1/4 cup cilantro, chopped

1 jalapeño, seeded and diced

1 lime, juiced

1/2 teaspoon honey

Method of Preparation:

1. Preheat the grill to medium-high heat.

2. Brush cod fillets with olive oil and season with Italian spice.

3. Grill cod fillets for 4-5 minutes per side, or until cooked through and flaky.

4. While the cod is grilling, prepare the mango salsa by combining diced mango, finely chopped red onion, chopped cilantro, diced jalapeño, lime juice, and honey in a bowl.

5. Mix well.

6. Serve grilled cod with mango salsa on top.

Spinach and Feta Stuffed Bell Peppers

Preparation Time: 30 minutes

Serves: 2

Calories: 180 **Sodium:** 50mg **Fats:** 10g **Carbs:** 15g **Cholesterol:** 10mg **Fiber:** 5g

Ingredients:

2 large bell peppers (any color), halved and seeds removed

1 tablespoon olive oil

2 cups fresh spinach leaves

1/4 cup diced onion

1 clove garlic, minced

1/4 cup crumbled low-fat cottage cheese

Method of Preparation:

1. Preheat the oven to 375°F (190°C).
2. Heat olive oil in a skillet over medium heat.
3. Add diced onion and minced garlic, and cook until softened.
4. Add fresh spinach leaves to the skillet and cook until wilted.
5. Remove the skillet from heat and stir in crumbled feta cheese.
6. Add desired spices.
7. Stuff each bell pepper half with the spinach and feta mixture.

8. Place stuffed bell peppers on a baking sheet lined with parchment paper.

9. Bake in the preheated oven for 20-25 minutes, or until the peppers are tender.

Shrimp and Vegetable Skewers with Brown Rice

Preparation Time: 20 minutes

Serves: 2

Calories: 180g **Sodium:** 30mg **Fats:** 8g **Carbs:** 3g **Cholesterol:** 70mg **Fiber:** 5g

Ingredients:

12 large shrimp, peeled and deveined

1 zucchini, sliced

1 bell pepper (any color), diced

1 onion, diced

1 tablespoon olive oil

Cooked brown rice, for serving

Method of Preparation:

1. Preheat the grill or grill pan to medium-high heat.

2. Thread shrimp, zucchini slices, bell pepper pieces, and diced onion onto skewers.

3. Brush skewers with olive oil and season with desired low sodium spices.

4. Grill skewers for 3-4 minutes per side, or until shrimp are pink and vegetables are tender.

5. Serve shrimp and vegetable skewers over cooked brown rice.

Baked Tilapia with Herb Crust

Preparation Time: 20 minutes

Serves: 2

Calories: 200g **Sodium:** 50mg **Fats:** 8g **Carbs:** 5g **Cholesterol:** 40mg **Fiber:** 1g

Ingredients:

2 tilapia fillets

2 tablespoons whole wheat breadcrumbs

1 tablespoon grated low-fat cheese

1 tablespoon chopped fresh parsley

1 tablespoon chopped fresh basil

1 tablespoon olive oil

1 lemon, sliced

Method of Preparation:

1. Preheat the oven to 400°F (200°C).
2. In a small bowl, combine whole wheat breadcrumbs, grated low-fat cheese, chopped fresh parsley, chopped fresh basil and olive oil to make the herb crust.
3. Place tilapia fillets on a baking sheet lined with parchment paper.
4. Spread the herb crust mixture evenly over the top of each tilapia fillet.
5. Place lemon slices on top of the herb crust.
6. Bake in the preheated oven for 12-15 minutes, or until the tilapia is cooked through and flakes easily with a fork.

Eggplant Parmesan with Whole Wheat Pasta

Preparation Time: 40 minutes

Serves: 2

Calories: 140g **Sodium:** 50mg **Fats:** 10g**Carbs:** 40g **Cholesterol:** 10mg **Fiber:** 12g

Ingredients:

1 large eggplant, sliced into rounds

1 cup whole wheat breadcrumbs

1/4 cup grated low-fat Parmesan cheese

1 teaspoon dried oregano

1 teaspoon dried basil

2 eggs, beaten

2 cups marinara sauce (store-bought or homemade, low-sodium)

8 oz whole wheat pasta

Fresh basil leaves for garnish (optional)

Method of Preparation:

1. Preheat the oven to 400°F (200°C).
2. In a shallow bowl, combine whole wheat breadcrumbs, grated low-fat Parmesan cheese, dried oregano, and dried basil.
3. Dip eggplant slices into beaten eggs, then coat with the breadcrumb mixture.
4. Place coated eggplant slices on a baking sheet lined with parchment paper.
5. Bake in the preheated oven for 20-25 minutes, or until the eggplant is tender and golden brown.
6. While the eggplant is baking, cook whole wheat pasta according to package instructions.
7. In a saucepan, heat marinara sauce over medium heat until warmed through.
8. Serve baked eggplant slices over whole wheat pasta, topped with marinara sauce.
9. Garnish with fresh basil leaves, if desired.

Turkey Meatballs with Marinara Sauce and Zucchini Noodles

Preparation Time: 40 minutes

Serves: 2

Calories: 150g **Sodium:** 40mg **Fats:** 15g **Carbs:** 20g **Cholesterol:** 40mg **Fiber:** 6g

Ingredients:

1 lb. ground turkey

1/4 cup whole wheat breadcrumbs

1/4 cup grated low-fat cheese

1 egg, beaten

1 teaspoon dried basil

1 teaspoon dried oregano

2 cups marinara sauce (store-bought or homemade, low-sodium)

2 medium zucchinis, spiralized into noodles

Fresh parsley for garnish (optional)

Method of Preparation:

1. Preheat the oven to 400°F (200°C).

2. In a mixing bowl, combine ground turkey, whole wheat breadcrumbs, grated low-fat cheese, beaten egg, dried basil, dried oregano, salt, and black pepper.

3. Mix until well combined.

4. Roll the turkey mixture into meatballs and place them on a baking sheet lined with parchment paper.

5. Bake in the preheated oven for 20-25 minutes, or until the meatballs are cooked through.

6. While the meatballs are baking, heat marinara sauce in a saucepan over medium heat until warmed through.

7. Spiralize zucchini into noodles using a spiralizer.

8. In a separate skillet, heat a small amount of olive oil over medium heat.

9. Add zucchini noodles and sauté for 2-3 minutes, or until tender.

10. Serve turkey meatballs over zucchini noodles, topped with marinara sauce.

11. Garnish with fresh parsley, if desired.

Baked Chicken Thighs with Sweet Potatoes and Brussels Sprouts

Preparation Time: 40 minutes

Serves: 2

Calories: 180g **Sodium:** 20mg **Fats:** 15g **Carbs:** 30g **Cholesterol:** 30mg **Fiber:** 6g

Ingredients:

2 bone-in, skinless chicken thighs

1 sweet potato, peeled and diced

1 cup Brussels sprouts, halved

1 tablespoon olive oil

1 teaspoon dried thyme

1 teaspoon smoked paprika

Method of Preparation:

1. Preheat the oven to 400°F (200°C).

2. Place diced sweet potatoes and halved Brussels sprouts on a baking sheet lined with parchment paper.

3. Drizzle olive oil over the vegetables and sprinkle with dried thyme, smoked paprika, salt, and black pepper.

4. Toss to coat evenly.

5. Arrange chicken thighs on the baking sheet with the vegetables.

6. Bake in the preheated oven for 25-30 minutes, or until the chicken is cooked through and the vegetables are tender.

7. Serve baked chicken thighs with sweet potatoes and Brussels sprouts.

DESSERTS

Mixed Berry Parfait

Preparation Time: 10 minutes

Serves: 2

Calories: 100g **Sodium:** 50mg **Fats:** 5g **Carbs:** 30g **Cholesterol:** 10mg **Fiber:** 6g

Ingredients:

1 cup mixed berries (such as strawberries, blueberries, raspberries)

1 cup low-fat Greek yogurt (unsweetened)

1/4 cup granola (unsweetened)

1 tablespoon honey (optional)

Method of Preparation:

1. Rinse the mixed berries and pat them dry with a paper towel.
2. If using strawberries, hull and slice them.
3. In serving glasses or bowls, layer low-fat Greek yogurt, mixed berries, and granola.
4. Repeat the layers until the glasses are filled, ending with a layer of mixed berries on top.
5. Drizzle honey over the top layer if desired.
6. Serve immediately as a healthy and delicious breakfast or snack.

Baked Apples with Cinnamon

Preparation Time: 30 minutes

Serves: 2

Calories: 150g **Sodium:** 0mg **Fats:** 0g **Carbs:** 40g **Cholesterol:** 0mg **Fiber:** 8g

Ingredients:

2 apples (such as Granny Smith or Honeycrisp)

1 tablespoon lemon juice

1 teaspoon ground cinnamon

1 tablespoon honey (optional)

Method of Preparation:

1. Preheat the oven to 375°F (190°C).
2. Core the apples and cut them into thick slices.
3. Place the apple slices in a baking dish and drizzle with lemon juice.
4. Sprinkle ground cinnamon over the apple slices.
5. If desired, drizzle honey over the apple slices for added sweetness.

6. Bake in the preheated oven for 20-25 minutes, or until the apples are tender.

7. Serve baked apples warm as a healthy dessert or snack option.

Chia Seed Pudding

Preparation Time: 5 minutes

Serves: 2

Calories: 150g **Sodium:** 50mg **Fats:** 8g **Carbs:** 15g **Cholesterol:** 0mg **Fiber:** 10g

Ingredients:

1/4 cup chia seeds

1 cup unsweetened almond milk (or any milk of choice)

1 tablespoon honey or maple syrup (optional)

1/2 teaspoon vanilla extract

Fresh fruit for topping (optional)

Method of Preparation:

1. In a mixing bowl, combine chia seeds, unsweetened almond milk, honey or maple syrup (if using), and vanilla extract.
2. Stir well to combine.
3. Cover the bowl and refrigerate for at least 2 hours or overnight, allowing the chia seeds to absorb the liquid and thicken.
4. Stir the chia seed pudding mixture well before serving.
5. Divide the pudding into serving bowls and top with fresh fruit if desired.
6. Serve chilled as a nutritious breakfast or snack option.

Banana-Oat Cookies

Preparation Time: 25 minutes

Serves: 2

Calories: 100g **Sodium:** 0mg **Fats:** 6g **Carbs:** 35g **Cholesterol:** 0mg **Fiber:** 5g

Ingredients:

2 ripe bananas, mashed

1 cup rolled oats

1/4 cup chopped nuts (such as walnuts or almonds)

1/4 cup raisins or dried cranberries

1 teaspoon cinnamon

1/2 teaspoon vanilla extract

Method of Preparation:

1. Preheat the oven to 350°F (175°C).
2. Line a baking sheet with parchment paper.
3. In a mixing bowl, combine mashed bananas, rolled oats, chopped nuts, raisins or dried cranberries, cinnamon, and vanilla extract.
4. Mix well until all ingredients are incorporated.
5. Drop a spoonful of the cookie dough onto the prepared baking sheet, spacing them apart.
6. Flatten each cookie slightly with the back of a spoon.
7. Bake in the preheated oven for 15-20 minutes, or until the cookies are golden brown and firm.

8. Allow the cookies to cool on the baking sheet for a few minutes before transferring them to a wire rack to cool completely.

Dark Chocolate-Dipped Strawberries

Preparation Time: 20 minutes

Serves: 2

Calories: 150g **Sodium:** 0mg **Fats:** 10g **Carbs:** 15g **Cholesterol:** 0mg **Fiber:** 3g

Ingredients:

1 cup dark chocolate chips

1 tablespoon coconut oil

10 large strawberries, washed and dried

Method of Preparation:

1. Line a baking sheet with parchment paper.
2. In a microwave-safe bowl, combine dark chocolate chips and coconut oil.

3. Microwave in 30-second intervals, stirring in between, until the chocolate is fully melted and smooth.

4. Dip each strawberry into the melted chocolate, allowing any excess chocolate to drip off.

5. Place the chocolate-dipped strawberries onto the prepared baking sheet.

6. Refrigerate the strawberries for 15-20 minutes, or until the chocolate is set.

Frozen Yogurt Bark

Preparation Time: 10 minutes

Serves: 2

Calories: 150g **Sodium:** 50mg **Fats:** 5g **Carbs:** 20g **Cholesterol:** 0mg **Fiber:** 3g

Ingredients:

1 cup low-fat Greek yogurt (unsweetened)

1 tablespoon honey or maple syrup

1/4 cup mixed berries (such as blueberries, raspberries, and strawberries), chopped

2 tablespoons granola (unsweetened)

Method of Preparation:

1. Line a baking sheet with parchment paper.

2. In a mixing bowl, combine low-fat Greek yogurt and honey or maple syrup.

3. Mix well.

4. Spread the Greek yogurt mixture evenly onto the prepared baking sheet, using a spatula to smooth it out.

5. Sprinkle chopped mixed berries and granola over the Greek yogurt layer.

6. Place the baking sheet in the freezer for 2-3 hours, or until the yogurt bark is frozen solid.

7. Once frozen, break the yogurt bark into pieces.

8. Enjoy these refreshing and nutritious frozen treats straight from the freezer.

SOUPS AND STEWS

Chicken and Vegetable Soup

Preparation Time: 40 minutes

Serves: 2

Calories: 150g **Sodium:** 30mg **Fats:** 5g **Carbs:** 15g **Cholesterol:** 20mg **Fiber:** 4g

Ingredients:

2 boneless, skinless chicken breasts, diced

4 cups low-sodium chicken broth

1 onion, diced

2 carrots, diced

2 celery stalks, diced

2 cloves garlic, minced

1 teaspoon dried thyme

1 teaspoon dried rosemary

2 cups spinach leaves

Fresh parsley for garnish (optional)

A pinch of salt and pepper

Method of Preparation:

1. In a large pot, heat olive oil over medium heat.

2. Add diced onion, minced garlic, diced carrots, and diced celery.

3. Sauté until softened.

4. Add diced chicken breasts to the pot and cook until lightly browned.

5. Pour in low-sodium chicken broth and add dried thyme and dried rosemary.

6. Bring to a boil.

7. Reduce heat to low and simmer for 20-25 minutes, or until the chicken is cooked through and vegetables are tender.

8. Stir in spinach leaves and cook until wilted.

9. Adjust seasoning with salt and black pepper if needed.

10. Serve hot, garnished with fresh parsley if desired.

Turkey and Quinoa Stew

Preparation Time: 40 minutes

Serves: 2

Calories: 100g **Sodium:** 40mg **Fats:** 8g **Carbs:** 25g
Cholesterol: 30mg **Fiber:** 5g

Ingredients:

1 lb. ground turkey

1 onion, diced

2 cloves garlic, minced

2 carrots, diced

2 celery stalks, diced

1 can (15 oz) diced tomatoes

1/2 cup quinoa, rinsed

4 cups low-sodium chicken broth

1 teaspoon dried thyme

1 teaspoon dried rosemary

Fresh parsley for garnish (optional)

A pinch of salt and black pepper

Method of Preparation:

1. In a large pot, cook ground turkey over medium heat until browned and cooked through.

2. Add diced onion and minced garlic to the pot, and cook until softened.

3. Add diced carrots, diced celery, diced tomatoes, rinsed quinoa, low-sodium chicken broth, dried thyme and dried rosemary to the pot.

4. Bring to a boil.

5. Reduce heat to low and simmer for 20-25 minutes, or until the quinoa is cooked and vegetables are tender.

6. Adjust seasoning with salt and black pepper if needed.

7. Serve hot, garnished with fresh parsley if desired.

Lentil Soup

Preparation Time: 45 minutes

Serves: 2

Calories: 120g **Sodium:** 30mg **Fats:** 2g **Carbs:** 35g **Cholesterol:** 0mg **Fiber:** 10g

Ingredients:

1 cup dried lentils, rinsed

4 cups low-sodium vegetable broth

1 onion, diced

2 carrots, diced

2 celery stalks, diced

2 cloves garlic, minced

1 teaspoon dried thyme

1 teaspoon ground cumin

Fresh parsley for garnish (optional)

Method of Preparation:

1. In a large pot, combine dried lentils, low-sodium vegetable broth, diced onion, diced carrots, diced celery, minced garlic, dried thyme, ground cumin, salt, and black pepper.
2. Bring to a boil.
3. Reduce heat to low and simmer for 25-30 minutes, or until the lentils are tender.
4. Adjust with desired spices if needed.
5. Serve hot, garnished with fresh parsley if desired.

Vegetable Barley Soup

Preparation Time: 45 minutes

Serves: 2

Calories: 100g **Sodium:** 30mg **Fats:** 3g **Carbs:** 35g
Cholesterol: 0mg **Fiber:** 8g

Ingredients:

1 tablespoon olive oil

1 onion, diced

2 carrots, diced

2 celery stalks, diced

2 cloves garlic, minced

1/2 cup pearl barley, rinsed

4 cups low-sodium vegetable broth

1 can (15 oz) diced tomatoes

1 teaspoon dried thyme

1 teaspoon dried rosemary

2 cups chopped spinach leaves

Fresh parsley for garnish (optional)

Method of Preparation:

1. In a large pot, heat olive oil over medium heat.
2. Add diced onion, diced carrots, diced celery, and minced garlic.
3. Sauté until softened.
4. Add rinsed pearl barley to the pot and cook for 1-2 minutes, stirring frequently.
5. Pour in low-sodium vegetable broth and add diced tomatoes (with their juices), dried thyme and dried rosemary.
6. Bring to a boil.
7. Reduce heat to low and simmer for 30-35 minutes, or until the barley is tender.
8. Stir in chopped spinach leaves and cook until wilted.
9. Adjust seasoning with salt and black pepper if needed.
10. Serve hot, garnished with fresh parsley if desired.

Minestrone Soup

Preparation Time: 30 minutes

Serves: 2

Calories: 150g **Sodium:** 40mg **Fats:** 3g **Carbs:** 45g
Cholesterol: 0mg **Fiber:** 10g

Ingredients:

1 tablespoon olive oil

1 onion, diced

2 carrots, diced

2 celery stalks, diced

2 cloves garlic, minced

1 can (15 oz) diced tomatoes

4 cups low-sodium vegetable broth

1 can (15 oz) kidney beans, drained and rinsed

1/2 cup small pasta (such as ditalini or small shells)

1 teaspoon dried basil

1 teaspoon dried oregano

2 cups chopped spinach leaves

Fresh parsley for garnish (optional)

Method of Preparation:

1. In a large pot, heat olive oil over medium heat.
2. Add diced onion, diced carrots, diced celery, and minced garlic.
3. Sauté until softened.
4. Add diced tomatoes (with their juices) to the pot and cook for 2-3 minutes.
5. Pour in low-sodium vegetable broth and add drained and rinsed kidney beans, small pasta, dried basil, dried oregano.
6. Bring to a boil.
7. Reduce heat to low and simmer for 15-20 minutes, or until the pasta is cooked through.
8. Stir in chopped spinach leaves and cook until wilted.
9. Adjust seasoning with salt and black pepper if needed.
10. Serve hot, garnished with fresh parsley if desired.

POULTRY MAINS

Herb-Roasted Turkey Breast

Preparation Time: 90 minutes

Serves: 2

Calories: 100g **Sodium:** 50mg **Fats:** 10g **Carbs:** 0g
Cholesterol: 20mg **Fiber:** 0g

Ingredients:

1 turkey breast (bone-in, skin-on), about 2 lbs.

2 tablespoons olive oil

1 tablespoon chopped fresh rosemary

1 tablespoon chopped fresh thyme

1 tablespoon chopped fresh parsley

2 cloves garlic, minced

1 lemon, sliced

Method of Preparation:

1. Preheat the oven to 375°F (190°C).

2. In a small bowl, mix together olive oil, chopped fresh rosemary, chopped fresh thyme, chopped fresh parsley and minced garlic to create the herb mixture.

3. Place the turkey breast on a roasting pan or baking dish.

4. Rub the herb mixture all over the turkey breast, making sure to coat it evenly.

5. Place lemon slices on top of the turkey breast.

6. Roast in the preheated oven for 60-75 minutes, or until the internal temperature reaches 165°F (74°C) when tested with a meat thermometer.

7. Once cooked, remove the turkey breast from the oven and let it rest for 10 minutes before slicing.

8. Serve hot, sliced thinly, and enjoy!

Lemon Rosemary Chicken Skewers

Preparation Time: 40 minutes

Serves: 2

Calories: 100g **Sodium:** 50mg **Fats:** 8g **Carbs:** 2g **Cholesterol:** 40mg **Fiber:** 0g

Ingredients:

2 boneless, skinless chicken breasts, cut into chunks

2 tablespoons olive oil

1 tablespoon chopped fresh rosemary

1 tablespoon chopped fresh thyme

2 cloves garlic, minced

Zest and juice of 1 lemon

Wooden skewers, soaked in water for 30 minutes

Method of Preparation:

1. In a bowl, mix together olive oil, chopped fresh rosemary, chopped fresh thyme, minced garlic, lemon zest and lemon juice to create the marinade.,

2. Add the chicken chunks to the marinade and toss to coat evenly.

3. Cover and refrigerate for at least 30 minutes, or up to 4 hours.

4. Preheat the grill or grill pan over medium-high heat.

5. Thread the marinated chicken chunks onto the soaked wooden skewers.

6. Grill the skewers for 6-8 minutes per side, or until the chicken is cooked through and golden brown.

7. Remove from the grill and let them rest for a few minutes before serving.

8. Serve hot, and enjoy these flavorful chicken skewers!

Poached Chicken with Herbs

Preparation Time: 25 minutes

Serves: 2

Calories: 150g **Sodium:** 20mg **Fats:** 3g **Carbs:** 0g **Cholesterol:** 40mg **Fiber:** 0g

Ingredients:

2 boneless, skinless chicken breasts

4 cups low-sodium chicken broth

2 cloves garlic, smashed

2 sprigs fresh rosemary

4 sprigs fresh thyme

Fresh parsley for garnish (optional)

Method of Preparation:

1. In a large saucepan, bring the chicken broth to a simmer over medium heat.

2. Add smashed garlic cloves, fresh rosemary sprigs, and fresh thyme sprigs to the simmering broth.

3. Season the chicken breasts with desired low sodium spices, then add them to the simmering broth.

4. Reduce heat to low, cover, and simmer for 15-20 minutes, or until the chicken is cooked through and no longer pink in the center.

5. Once cooked, remove the chicken breasts from the poaching liquid and let them rest for a few minutes before slicing.

6. Serve the poached chicken hot, garnished with fresh parsley if desired.

7. Enjoy this tender and flavorful chicken dish!

Ginger Soy Glazed Chicken Thighs

Preparation Time: 40 minutes

Serves: 2

Calories: 150g **Sodium:** 40mg **Fats:** 20g **Carbs:** 10g **Cholesterol:** 20mg **Fiber:** 0g

Ingredients:

4 bone-in, skin-on chicken thighs

2 tablespoons low-sodium soy sauce

1 tablespoon honey

1 tablespoon grated fresh ginger

2 cloves garlic, minced

1 tablespoon sesame oil

1 teaspoon rice vinegar

1 green onion, thinly sliced for garnish (optional)

Sesame seeds for garnish (optional)

Method of Preparation:

1. In a small bowl, whisk together low-sodium soy sauce, honey, grated fresh ginger, minced garlic, sesame oil, and rice vinegar to create the marinade.

2. Place chicken thighs in a shallow dish and pour the marinade over them, ensuring they are evenly coated.

Cover and refrigerate for at least 30 minutes, or up to 4 hours.

3. Preheat the oven to 400°F (200°C).

4. Place marinated chicken thighs on a baking sheet lined with parchment paper.

5. Bake in the preheated oven for 25-30 minutes, or until the chicken is cooked through and the glaze is caramelized.

6. Garnish with thinly sliced green onions and sesame seeds, if desired.

Mediterranean Chicken Salad with Olives and Feta

Preparation Time: 20 minutes

Serves: 2

Calories: 100g **Sodium:** 40mg **Fats:** 15g **Carbs:** 10g **Cholesterol:** 80mg **Fiber:** 3g

Ingredients:

2 boneless, skinless chicken breasts

2 cups mixed salad greens

1/4 cup Kalamata olives, pitted and halved

1/4 cup crumbled low-fat cottage cheese

1/4 cup cherry tomatoes, halved

2 tablespoons extra virgin olive oil

1 tablespoon balsamic vinegar

1 teaspoon dried oregano

Method of Preparation:

1. Season chicken breasts with dried oregano and desired low sodium spices.
2. Heat a grill or grill pan over medium-high heat.
3. Grill chicken breasts for 6-8 minutes per side, or until cooked through.
4. Let the chicken rest for a few minutes, then slice into strips.
5. In a large bowl, toss mixed salad greens, Kalamata olives, crumbled low-fat cottage cheese, and cherry tomatoes.
6. Drizzle extra virgin olive oil and balsamic vinegar over the salad, and toss to coat evenly.

7. Divide the salad onto serving plates and top with sliced grilled chicken.

8. Serve immediately as a refreshing and flavorful meal.

SEAFOOD MAINS

Oven-Roasted Mahi Mahi with Pineapple Salsa

Preparation Time: 20 minutes

Serves: 2

Calories: 150g **Sodium:** 20mg **Fats:** 10g **Carbs:** 15g **Cholesterol:** 20mg **Fiber:** 2g

Ingredients:

2 Mahi Mahi fillets

1 tablespoon olive oil

1 teaspoon paprika

1 teaspoon garlic powder

1/2 teaspoon cumin

Pineapple Salsa:

1 cup diced pineapple

1/4 cup diced red bell pepper

1/4 cup diced red onion

2 tablespoons chopped fresh cilantro

Juice of 1 lime

Method of Preparation:

1. Preheat the oven to 400°F (200°C).
2. In a small bowl, mix together olive oil, paprika, garlic powder, cumin.
3. Place Mahi Mahi fillets on a baking sheet lined with parchment paper.
4. Brush the spice mixture over the fillets.
5. Bake in the preheated oven for 12-15 minutes, or until the fish is cooked through and flakes easily with a fork.
6. While the fish is baking, prepare the pineapple salsa by combining diced pineapple, diced red bell pepper, diced red onion, chopped fresh cilantro, lime juice, salt, and black pepper in a bowl.

7. Mix well.

8. Serve the oven-roasted Mahi Mahi hot, topped with pineapple salsa.

Garlic Butter Lobster Tails

Preparation Time: 20 minutes

Serves: 2

Calories: 100g **Sodium:** 30mg **Fats:** 20g **Carbs:** 2g **Cholesterol:** 10mg **Fiber:** 0g

Ingredients:

2 lobster tails

4 tablespoons unsalted butter, melted

2 cloves garlic, minced

1 tablespoon chopped fresh parsley

Lemon wedges for serving

Method of Preparation:

1. Preheat the oven to 375°F (190°C).

2. Using kitchen shears, cut along the top of the lobster tails to expose the meat.

3. Gently lift the meat and place it on top of the shell.

4. In a small bowl, mix together melted butter, minced garlic, chopped fresh parsley, salt, and black pepper.

5. Brush the garlic butter mixture over the lobster tails, ensuring they are evenly coated.

6. Place the lobster tails on a baking sheet lined with parchment paper.

7. Bake in the preheated oven for 12-15 minutes, or until the lobster meat is opaque and cooked through.

8. Serve hot with lemon wedges on the side.

9. Enjoy these succulent garlic butter lobster tails!

Blackened Catfish with Avocado Corn Salsa

Preparation Time: 15 minutes

Serves: 2

Calories: 150g **Sodium:** 40mg **Fats:** 15g **Carbs:** 20g **Cholesterol:** 30mg **Fiber:** 6g

Ingredients:

2 catfish fillets

1 tablespoon olive oil

1 tablespoon blackening seasoning

A pinch of salt

Avocado Corn Salsa:

1 avocado, diced

1/2 cup corn kernels (fresh or frozen, thawed)

1/4 cup diced red onion

1/4 cup diced red bell pepper

1 tablespoon chopped fresh cilantro

Juice of 1 lime

Method of Preparation:

1. Rub catfish fillets with olive oil and sprinkle blackening seasoning and salt on both sides.
2. Heat a skillet over medium-high heat.
3. Once hot, add catfish fillets to the skillet.
4. Cook for 3-4 minutes per side, or until the fish is blackened and cooked through.

5. While the fish is cooking, prepare the avocado corn salsa by combining diced avocado, corn kernels, diced red onion, diced red bell pepper, chopped fresh cilantro and lime juice in a bowl. Mix well.

6. Serve blackened catfish hot, topped with avocado corn salsa.

Spicy Thai Coconut Shrimp Soup

Preparation Time: 30 minutes

Serves: 2

Calories: 300g **Sodium:** 400mg **Fats:** 20g **Carbs:** 10g **Cholesterol:** 150mg **Fiber:** 2g

Ingredients:

1 tablespoon coconut oil

1 onion, diced

2 cloves garlic, minced

1 tablespoon grated fresh ginger

1 red bell pepper, sliced

1 green bell pepper, sliced

1 can (13.5 oz) coconut milk

4 cups low-sodium chicken broth

1 tablespoon Thai red curry paste

1 tablespoon fish sauce

1 tablespoon lime juice

1 pound shrimp, peeled and deveined

Fresh cilantro for garnish (optional)

Method of Preparation:

1. In a large pot, heat coconut oil over medium heat. Add diced onion, minced garlic, and grated fresh ginger.
2. Sauté until fragrant.
3. Add sliced red bell pepper and green bell pepper to the pot and cook until softened.
4. Pour in coconut milk and low-sodium chicken broth. Stir in Thai red curry paste, fish sauce, and lime juice. Bring to a simmer.

5. Add peeled and deveined shrimp to the pot and cook for 3-4 minutes, or until the shrimp is pink and cooked through.

6. Serve the spicy Thai coconut shrimp soup hot, garnished with fresh cilantro if desired.

Pan-Seared Sea Bass with Lemon Caper Sauce

Preparation Time: 15 minutes

Serves: 2

Calories: 150g **Sodium:** 30mg **Fats:** 25g **Carbs:** 2g **Cholesterol:** 50mg **Fiber:** 0g

Ingredients:

2 sea bass fillets

2 tablespoons olive oil

Lemon Caper Sauce:

2 tablespoons unsalted butter

2 tablespoons capers, drained

Juice of 1 lemon

1 tablespoon chopped fresh parsley

Method of Preparation:

1. Season sea bass fillets with desired low sodium spices on both sides.

2. Heat olive oil in a skillet over medium-high heat. Once hot, add sea bass fillets to the skillet.

3. Cook for 4-5 minutes per side, or until the fish is golden brown and cooked through.

4. While the fish is cooking, prepare the lemon caper sauce by melting unsalted butter in a small saucepan over medium heat.

5. Add drained capers, lemon juice, chopped fresh parsley, salt, and black pepper.

6. Cook for 1-2 minutes, stirring occasionally.

7. Serve pan-seared sea bass hot, topped with lemon caper sauce.

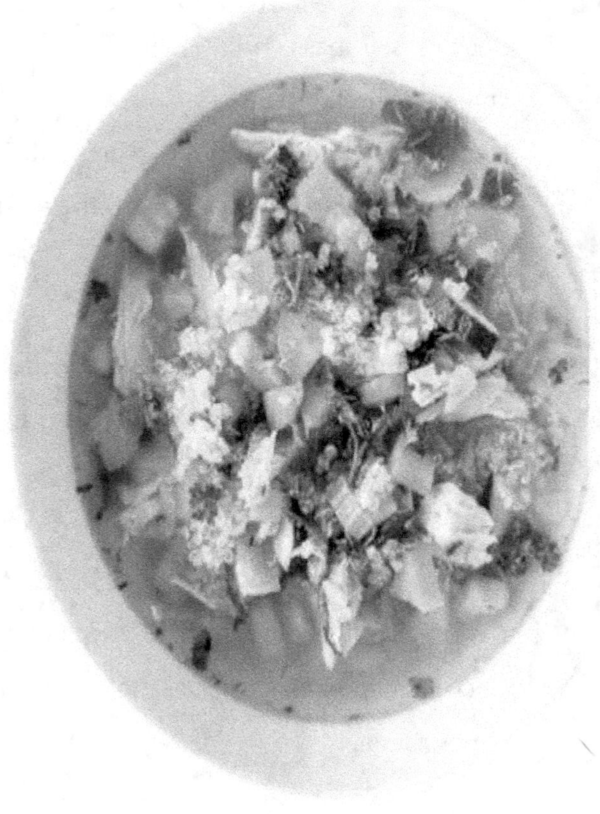

CONCLUSION

In conclusion, this cookbook is a valuable resource for you seeking to manage your condition through nutrition.

By focusing on heart-healthy foods that support overall cardiovascular health and reduce the risk of complications, such a cookbook can empower individuals with AFib to take control of their health and well-being.

Throughout this cookbook, I emphasized the importance of a balanced diet rich in fruits, vegetables, whole grains, lean proteins, and healthy fats.

These foods provide essential nutrients, vitamins, and minerals that are beneficial for heart health and can help manage AFib symptoms.

Additionally, I have highlighted the importance of limiting or avoiding certain foods and beverages that can trigger AFib episodes or worsen symptoms.

These include foods high in sodium, saturated fats, cholesterol, and added sugars, as well as caffeinated and alcoholic beverages.

By following the recipes and meal plans provided in this cookbook, you can create delicious and nutritious meals that support their heart health and overall well-being.

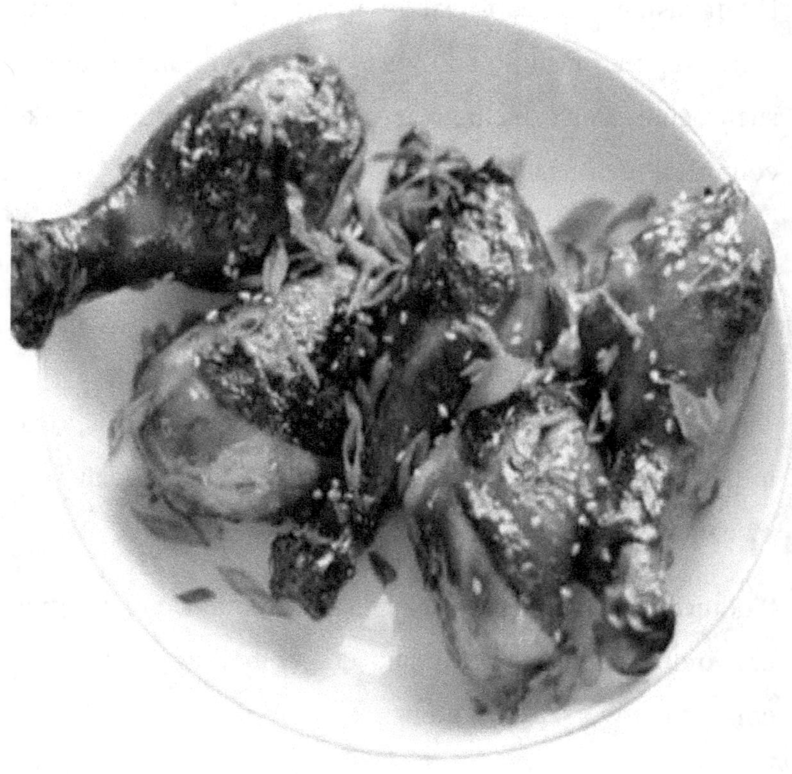